Table of Contents

Introduction: Embarking on a Nutritional Odyssey

Unleash the Potential of Superfoods

We all understand the importance of healthy foods like fruits, vegetables, and nuts. But with countless options, wouldn't it be simpler to have a curated list of superfoods that can transform your health? Imagine having a user-friendly guide to help you lead a more vibrant life. Well, you're in luck because we've gathered a selection of nine remarkable superfoods to kickstart your journey to a healthier you. These superfoods, along with 14 others, are featured in the book "Superfoods Health-Style" by Steven G. Pratt, M.D.

1. Apples: Your Heart's Ally Apples aren't just tasty; they're also heart-healthy. They lower the risk of heart disease, cancer, high blood pressure, and type 2 diabetes. Remember, don't discard the peel; it's loaded with antioxidants. An apple a day truly does work wonders for your health!

2. Avocados: Nature's Nutrient Booster Looking to maximize nutrient absorption from your meals? Avocados are the answer. Their healthy fats enhance nutrient absorption. Plus, avocados are satisfying and can assist with weight management. Enjoy half an avocado two to three times weekly.

3. Dark Chocolate: Sweetness with Benefits Indulge in dark chocolate guilt-free. It's not only delicious but also packed with polyphenols that reduce blood pressure and combat inflammation. A little daily treat of dark chocolate (not milk chocolate) can have a positive impact on your health.

4. Olive Oil: Liquid Gold for Well-being Olive oil, a Mediterranean diet staple, lowers the risk of cancer, high blood pressure, and heart disease. Choose a daily tablespoon of extra virgin olive oil with high polyphenol content for maximum benefits.

5. Garlic: Heart Health Hero Garlic, like its cousin onion, is a cardiovascular superstar. Regular consumption lowers blood pressure, triglycerides, and LDL cholesterol. For the full health benefits, opt for fresh garlic, either raw or cooked.

6. Honey: Nature's Sweet Medicine Don't underestimate the power of honey. It boosts antioxidants, aids digestion, and reduces cholesterol and blood pressure. When you need an energy boost, choose honey over sugar. It stabilizes blood sugar and energy levels. Opt for dark honey for extra antioxidants.

7. Kiwis: The Vitamin C and E Boost Kiwis are bursting with vitamins C and E, which reduce asthma, osteoarthritis, colon cancer risk, and boost immunity. Get your vitamin E without extra calories found in nuts and oils. Consume one kiwi two to three times a week.

8. Onions: Versatile Sibling of Garlic Onions share numerous benefits with garlic, including promoting cardiovascular health and reducing inflammation. Use onions in your meals at least three times a week, and let them sit for a few minutes after cutting to maximize heart benefits.

9. Pomegranates: Potent Health Boosters Pomegranates are rich in phytochemicals like potassium, which lowers blood pressure, and they may slow prostate cancer and reduce atherosclerosis risk. Opt for 100% pomegranate juice, but avoid added sugar. Four to eight ounces several times a week can make a meaningful difference.

Why struggle with complex dietary choices when you can effortlessly enjoy the benefits of these superfoods? Embrace these nutritional powerhouses and embark on a journey to a healthier, more vibrant you.

Chapter 1: Nutritional Powerhouses: Unveiling the Superfoods

Are you ready to embark on a journey that will transform your health and vitality? In this chapter, we'll dive deep into the world of superfoods, those remarkable dietary heroes that hold the key to a healthier, more vibrant you. Imagine a life where you not only enjoy your meals but also fortify your body against diseases and aging. Buckle up as we uncover the extraordinary benefits of these nutritional powerhouses that have earned the unanimous approval of health experts worldwide.

1. Cantaloupe: A Vision Booster

Step into the world of cantaloupe, the unsung hero of vision enhancement. Discover how a mere quarter of this succulent fruit can supply your daily dose of vitamin A, potentially reducing the risk of cataracts. But that's just the beginning. Dive deeper to unravel the treasure trove of nutrients within cantaloupe, including vitamin C, B6, dietary fiber, and more. Learn how these elements bolster heart health, maintain blood sugar levels, and fortify your body against various diseases.

2. Blueberries: The Antioxidant Marvel

Blueberries, nature's antioxidant marvels, take the stage next. Delve into their world and uncover their sweet yet tangy secret. These tiny berries are not just a delight for your taste buds but also powerful warriors against cancer-causing free radicals. Learn how their low-calorie content masks a high concentration of anthocyanidins, amplifying the effects of vitamin C. Discover how they shield your body from a multitude of diseases.

3. Tomatoes: Heart and Cancer Defense

Tomatoes, with their luscious red hue, are not only a culinary delight but also potent defenders against heart disease and various cancers. Uncover the vitamins C, A, and K packed within these humble fruits and how they contribute to reducing blood clotting. Dive into the realm of tomato options, including the benefits of choosing organic varieties.

4. Sweet Potatoes: Nature's Lung Protector

Sweet potatoes, often overlooked, hold the key to robust health. Explore their impressive array of vitamins, including A and C, and discover how they play a vital role in lung health. Learn how these nutrient-rich tubers can be a boon for smokers and those exposed to second-hand smoke.

5. Spinach and Kale: The Ultimate Greens

Spinach and kale, the ultimate green superheroes, are next in line. These greens are not only cancer fighters but also guardians of your heart. Unearth their abundance of vitamins A, C, and calcium, and learn how they contribute to bone health and overall well-being.

6. Whole Grains: The Fiber Heroes

Whole grains step into the spotlight, champions of fiber and cancer-fighting wheat bran. Explore the world of whole-grain bread and pasta, and understand why they are your allies in preserving essential nutrients. Learn the stark difference between whole grains and their refined counterparts.

7. Walnuts: Omega-3 Warriors

Enter the world of walnuts, the omega-3-rich warriors that support your heart and brain. Discover the numerous benefits of these nuts, from cardiovascular protection to enhanced cognitive function.

8. Black Beans and Lentils: Fiber Friends

Black beans and lentils, your fiber friends, make an appearance. These legumes are your allies in maintaining stable blood sugar levels and promoting heart health. Explore how they provide quality protein without expanding your waistline.

9. Skim Milk and Yogurt: Bone Builders

Skim milk and yogurt step into the limelight as bone builders. Dive into the realm of calcium, vitamin D, and vitamin K, and understand how these dairy products protect against various conditions, including obesity and migraines.

10. Salmon: Heart-Healthy Protein

Finally, we delve into the world of salmon, the heart-healthy superstar rich in protein and omega-3 fats. Learn about the importance of choosing wild-caught salmon and discover why it's a wise choice for your overall health.

Green Tea and "Power" Water: Liquid Health

As we wrap up this chapter, we explore the liquid heroes that complement our superfood lineup. Green tea, with its antioxidant-rich profile and lower caffeine content, offers a multitude of health benefits. Additionally, we discuss the importance of staying hydrated with vitamin-packed water and naturally sweetened fruit-infused options.

Conclusion

As we conclude our journey through these top ten superfoods, remember that they are not just nutritious but life-changing. By embracing these foods, you are investing in your health and savoring the taste of a brighter, healthier future. Stay with us as we continue this journey to unlock the full potential of superfoods and unleash a healthier, more vibrant you.

Chapter 2: The Mirroring Effect: You Are What You Consume

Unlock the Power of Superfoods for Vibrant Health

In a world filled with dietary choices, a remarkable revelation has emerged in the realm of nutrition—a revelation that unveils a select group of 14 extraordinary foods, celebrated for their exceptional ability to elevate overall health. These foods, aptly christened "superfoods," stand out as nutritional powerhouses, offering a tantalizing combination of fewer calories, heightened levels of essential vitamins and minerals, and a treasury of disease-fighting antioxidants.

The 14 Nutritional Powerhouses

Beans (Legumes): These humble legumes punch above their weight, providing a wealth of essential nutrients. Rich in protein, fiber, vitamins, and minerals, they are known to promote heart health, manage blood sugar levels, and support weight management.

Berries (with a Special Nod to Blueberries): Bursting with flavor and nutrition, berries, especially blueberries, are packed with antioxidants and vitamins. They are champions in combating oxidative stress, enhancing brain function, and promoting heart health.

Broccoli: This cruciferous vegetable boasts an impressive array of vitamins, minerals, and antioxidants. Known for its potential to reduce the risk of chronic diseases, including cancer, broccoli is a versatile and nutrient-dense addition to your diet.

Green Tea: Renowned for its exceptional health benefits, green tea is rich in antioxidants called catechins. It supports weight management, improves brain function, and may lower the risk of various diseases, making it a staple in many healthy diets.

Nuts (with a Spotlight on Walnuts): Walnuts, in particular, are omega-3-rich superstars. They promote heart health, support brain function, and provide a satisfying dose of healthy fats and nutrients.

Oranges: Bursting with vitamin C, oranges are celebrated for their immune-boosting properties. They also provide a range of vitamins and minerals that contribute to overall health.

Pumpkin: This vibrant vegetable is a nutritional powerhouse, offering a wealth of vitamins, minerals, and antioxidants. It supports eye health, boosts immunity, and may even aid in weight loss.

Salmon: A rich source of omega-3 fatty acids, salmon is a heart-healthy choice. It promotes cardiovascular well-being, supports brain function, and provides essential nutrients for overall health.

Soy: As a plant-based protein, soy is a versatile superfood. It may lower the risk of chronic diseases, support bone health, and offer a valuable protein source for vegetarians and vegans.

Spinach: Packed with vitamins, minerals, and antioxidants, spinach is a nutritional powerhouse. It supports bone health, aids in managing blood pressure, and enhances overall vitality.

Tomatoes: Tomatoes are not only delicious but also offer an array of health benefits. Rich in vitamins C, A, and K, they are known to reduce the risk of heart disease and certain cancers.

Turkey: A lean source of protein, turkey is a dietary choice that supports muscle health, aids in weight management, and provides essential nutrients for overall well-being.

Whole Grains and Oats: These fiber-rich foods are the heroes of heart health. They help manage cholesterol levels, regulate blood sugar, and provide sustained energy.

Yogurt: A probiotic-rich dairy product, yogurt is beneficial for gut health and digestion. It provides essential nutrients like calcium, vitamin D, and protein.

The Superfood Advantage

The remarkable potential of these superfoods doesn't stop at combating diseases; it extends to enhancing overall well-being. These nutritional powerhouses recognize that every aspect of our body is interconnected, and they work harmoniously to optimize our health.

Embracing Superfoods for Lasting Transformation

By making these 14 superfoods the cornerstone of your balanced diet, you may find that weight loss trends and transient programs become a thing of the past. These foods offer a sustainable path to lasting transformation, where vibrant health becomes your daily reality.

The Consequences of an Imbalanced Diet

On the flip side, the repercussions of an imbalanced diet are extensive and far-reaching. Symptoms such as low energy levels, mood swings, persistent fatigue, and weight fluctuations serve as warning signs that your dietary choices may be askew.

Malnutrition: A Silent Threat

Malnutrition, often underestimated, can silently wreak havoc on your health. Depleted energy, irritability, a weakened immune system, and mineral deficiencies are just a few of the symptoms that may surface.

The Intricate Connection Between Body and Spirit

Recognizing the profound connection between body and spirit is an essential step on your journey to optimal health. An unhealthy body often leads to an unhealthy spirit. Conversely, nourishing our bodies with superfoods and nutrient-rich fresh foods invigorates not only our physical selves but also nurtures our spirits.

Modern Diets and the Nutrient Gap

In a world where modern diets heavily rely on prepackaged convenience foods, a concerning nutrient gap has emerged. Essential vitamins and minerals are often missing from our daily intake, leading to a significant impact on our mental faculties. Irritability, confusion, and a perpetual mental fog become unwelcome companions.

Superfoods: A Compelling Solution

Enter superfoods—a compelling solution that bridges the nutrient gap. They form the foundation for sound health and serve as a potent nutritional remedy to address an array of ailments and more. These extraordinary foods possess the power to rejuvenate your body, sharpen your mind, and uplift your spirit.

Unlocking the Potential of Superfoods

Join us on this transformative journey as we unlock the potential of these extraordinary foods. Through their vibrant flavors and exceptional benefits, they invite you to embrace a brighter, healthier future. With superfoods as your allies, you embark on a path to rejuvenate your body, empower your mind, and nurture your spirit. Welcome to the world of superfoods—where vibrant well-being awaits.

Chapter 3: Vibrant Health Through Colors: A Palette of Superfoods

Vibrant Health Through Colors: A Palette of Superfoods

Imagine a world where the colors of your plate are not just visually appealing but also brimming with vibrant health. This is the world of superfoods, where nature's palette offers a rainbow of nutrients and benefits. In this chapter, we delve into the captivating realm of colorful superfoods that hold the key to unlocking your body's full potential. These foods aren't just visually appealing; they are nutritional powerhouses, each hue representing a unique set of vitamins, minerals, and antioxidants that can enhance your well-being.

Red: The Radiant Hue of Health

The color red signifies not only love but also vitality and energy. In the realm of superfoods, red foods like tomatoes, strawberries, and watermelon are rich in lycopene—an antioxidant known for its heart-protective qualities. Dive into the world of crimson and discover how these red wonders can safeguard your cardiovascular health and invigorate your life.

Orange: A Burst of Sunshine in Every Bite

The vibrant hue of orange conjures images of sunsets and warmth. But did you know that orange superfoods like carrots, sweet potatoes, and oranges themselves offer a burst of sunshine for your health? Packed with beta-carotene, a precursor to vitamin A, these foods promote healthy skin, boost your immune system, and may even reduce the risk of certain cancers. Let's explore how the color orange can illuminate your path to vibrant health.

Yellow: The Golden Glow of Vitality

Yellow superfoods, including bananas, pineapples, and corn, radiate the golden glow of vitality. Rich in essential nutrients like potassium, vitamin C, and folate, they contribute to your overall well-being. Discover the sunshine within yellow foods as we unravel their potential to enhance your mood, support your heart, and fortify your immune system.

Green: Nature's Elixir for Life

Green foods, such as spinach, broccoli, and kale, embody the essence of nature's elixir for life. Bursting with chlorophyll, vitamins, and minerals, these superfoods are a beacon of health. Join us on a journey through lush green fields as we explore how these verdant wonders can detoxify your body, boost your energy, and promote vibrant longevity.

Blue and Purple: The Mystique of Antioxidant Power

The mysterious allure of blue and purple superfoods, like blueberries, blackberries, and eggplants, lies in their antioxidant power. Anthocyanins, the compounds responsible for their captivating colors, are also known for their ability to combat oxidative stress. Dive into the world of these enigmatic foods and uncover their potential to enhance brain function, protect your cells, and fight inflammation.

White: The Purity of Nutrient-Rich Superfoods

White may symbolize purity, and when it comes to superfoods like cauliflower, garlic, and mushrooms, it signifies the purity of nutrient-rich goodness. Despite their unassuming appearance, white superfoods are brimming with vitamins, minerals, and unique compounds that support your immune system, promote heart health, and even possess cancer-fighting properties. Join us as we unravel the secrets of these humble yet potent foods.

The Colorful Superfood Advantage

As we explore the vibrant world of colorful superfoods, you'll gain a deeper understanding of how each hue represents a wealth of health benefits. By incorporating a spectrum of colors into your diet, you'll not only savor a variety of flavors but also nourish your body with a diverse range of nutrients. Join us on this colorful journey as we unlock the potential of nature's palette to rejuvenate your body, uplift your spirit, and embark on a path to vibrant well-being.

Chapter 4: Age-Defying Elegance: Unleashing the Beauty of Superfoods

Unlocking Ageless Beauty with Nature's Superfoods

Embark on a journey into the realm of age-defying beauty with nature's most potent superfoods. These treasures offer more than just nutrition; they are your allies in revealing your timeless allure.

Goji Berries: The Secret of Youthful Radiance Often celebrated as the "Fountain of Youth," goji berries are true nutritional gems. They transcend mere sustenance and become your companions in the quest for enduring beauty. Originating in Tibet, these vibrant red berries are packed with vitamins, minerals, amino acids, phytochemicals, and essential fatty acids, making them deserving of their anti-aging reputation. The incredible health benefits of goji berries are diverse. They strengthen the immune system, lower cholesterol levels, support eye health, and even have mood-enhancing and weight loss properties due to their rich nutrient profile. What sets goji berries apart is their exceptional vitamin content: 500 times more vitamin C than oranges, surpassing carrot's beta-carotene levels, and a partnership with vitamin E and essential fatty acids, creating a powerful elixir for anti-aging and radiant beauty. Dive deeper, and you'll find polysaccharides stimulating the secretion of rejuvenating human growth hormone, along with a rich blend of B vitamins, 21 essential minerals, and 18 amino acids. A remarkable testament to the power of goji berries is the story of Li Qing Yuen, who reportedly consumed them daily and lived an astonishing 252 years. These small red wonders offer benefits beyond their size.

Aloe Vera: Nature's Collagen Boost When it comes to achieving youthful, wrinkle-free skin, Aloe Vera takes center stage. This miracle plant has the remarkable ability to enhance collagen production naturally, offering a compelling alternative to invasive cosmetic procedures. Aloe Vera boasts a wealth of over 200 active compounds, including 20 essential minerals, 18 amino acids, and even the rare vitamin B12. Its natural antimicrobial properties combat fungi and bacteria, while anti-inflammatory plant steroids and enzymes soothe the skin. Beyond its benefits for the skin, Aloe Vera aids in digestion, bolsters the immune system, and excels at healing, moisturizing, and rejuvenating the skin by stimulating collagen production. You can savor Aloe Vera in its freshest form by simply scraping out the inner gel and blending it with fruits to create a beauty-boosting smoothie. Its versatility in skincare and health makes Aloe Vera a true gift from nature.

Avocados: Nature's Skin Softener Avocados, with their creamy texture and rich taste, are not just a culinary delight; they are a gift to your skin. Their unique composition allows them to be readily absorbed, infusing your complexion with a delightful softness and suppleness that's hard to match. What makes avocados exceptional for your skin is their rich content of vitamin E, antioxidant carotenoids, and the master antioxidant glutathione. Glutathione, in particular, plays a crucial role in combating pollutants like cigarette smoke and UV radiation, making it a formidable defender against premature aging. The benefits of avocados extend beyond skin deep. They hold promise in various health domains, from cancer prevention to heart disease management. So, the next time you enjoy a serving of avocado toast or guacamole, know that you're not just savoring a delicious treat; you're indulging in a natural elixir for radiant skin and overall well-being.

Chlorella: The Cellular Fountain of Youth Chlorella, often referred to as the "Cellular Fountain of Youth," is a microscopic green algae rich in nucleic acids RNA, and DNA. These molecules are the blueprints for your body's growth, repair, and efficient nutrient utilization. As we age, our bodies produce fewer nucleic acids, and this decline is associated with premature aging and weakened immunity. Research has shown that chlorella supplements can help replenish RNA and DNA, promoting overall health, immunity, and longevity. It's not just about nucleic acids; chlorella is a treasure trove of vitamins, minerals, antioxidants, enzymes, and amino acids. In his book 'Healing with Whole Foods,' Paul Pitchford recognizes chlorella for its role in preventing premature aging and boosting immunity. It's a superfood that truly nourishes your cells from the inside out.

Bee Pollen: Nature's Skin Elixir Bee pollen, often called "Nature's Skin Elixir," is a remarkable substance for achieving youthful and radiant skin. Renowned dermatologist Dr. Lars-Erik Essen successfully treats various skin conditions, including acne, with bee pollen. His findings highlight the remarkable effects of bee pollen on skin health, attributed to its ability to prevent premature aging of skin cells, stimulate the growth of new skin tissue, and improve blood circulation to skin cells. What sets bee pollen apart is its high concentration of nucleic acids RNA and DNA, which are vital for cell health and regeneration. Additionally, bee pollen exhibits natural antibiotic properties and is packed with essential nutrients. Beyond its beautifying powers, bee pollen offers a myriad of health benefits. It fights infections, lowers cholesterol levels, strengthens the blood, boosts immunity, enhances stamina, promotes longevity, and has even been linked to increased libido. This small yet potent substance is a true gem from nature.

Coconut Oil: The Metabolism Booster Coconut oil, celebrated for its metabolism-boosting properties, is also a remarkable beauty elixir. It contains antioxidants that safeguard your skin from free radical damage, effectively preserving its youthfulness. Whether used internally or externally, coconut oil proves to be a reliable ally in skincare. It is enriched with lauric acid, a potent antimicrobial fatty acid that battles bacteria, viruses, and fungi, making it an ideal choice for skin health. Additionally, it can accelerate metabolism, aiding in weight management and overall vitality.

By embracing these nature-derived superfoods, you're not just nourishing your body from the inside out; you're also unlocking age-defying beauty the natural way.

Chapter 5: The Fountain of Youth: Superfoods for Longevity

Unlocking the Secrets of Food: Your Body's Natural Defense

Recent groundbreaking research has unveiled a captivating relationship between certain chemicals in our foods and our unique genetic makeup. This discovery holds the tantalizing potential to unleash our body's natural defense mechanisms, effectively thwarting the perils of cancer, cardiovascular disease, and premature aging. It paints a picture of a future where we can precisely identify genetic predispositions to diseases and tailor our diets accordingly. Imagine a world where we know precisely which foods to embrace and which to shun, actively thwarting genetic maladies before they take hold. While that future beckons, there's a wealth of knowledge available today that empowers us to age gracefully and healthily.

Lycopene: The Heart of Red

Now, let's delve into the vibrant world of lycopene, the brilliant pigment that paints tomatoes red. Beyond its vivid hue, lycopene emerges as a potent ally against some of the most prevalent health concerns of our time. This remarkable compound has been associated with reducing the risk of cardiovascular disease, select cancers, and even macular degeneration. But lycopene's benefits don't end there; it also bestows greater self-sufficiency upon the elderly, making it a true champion for aging populations.

While fresh tomatoes certainly have their merits, the most absorbable forms of lycopene are found within cooked tomato products like spaghetti sauce, soup, and prepared salsas. And the good news is, it doesn't stop at tomatoes. Other foods like pink grapefruit, guava, red bell peppers, and watermelon also boast this extraordinary compound, inviting us to diversify our diets while reaping the health rewards.

Orange Bounty: Beta-Carotene Riches

Enter the vibrant world of orange-hued fruits, which beckon with beta-carotene, the precursor to vitamin A. Embracing at least two cups of these orange treasures, such as sweet potatoes, squash, and carrots, fortifies your skin, supports your vision, and potentially shields against a range of health concerns, including cancers, cardiovascular diseases, and osteoporosis.

But the beta-carotene story doesn't end there. Lutein and lycopene, also found in these orange gems, hold the keys to safeguarding your vision, protecting your skin from sun damage, and potentially diminishing the visible signs of aging. In this nutritional orchestra, mangos and cantaloupes stand proudly among the beta-carotene-rich cadre, inviting you to savor their delicious and healthful offerings.

Emerald Elixir: The Power of Greens

Now, let's turn our attention to the often-unsung heroes in your culinary repertoire: dark leafy greens. These emerald wonders are the guardians of your heart health, significantly reducing the risk of cardiovascular disease while potentially preserving your eyesight. Dietary guidelines beckon us to savor at least three cups of greens weekly, whether fresh, frozen, or conveniently bagged. The versatility of these greens opens a world of culinary possibilities, inviting you to incorporate them into your meals for both their taste and their unparalleled health benefits.

Omega-3 Fatty Acids: Nourishing Your Brain

Aging isn't just about the body; it profoundly affects your mind too. Here, the spotlight falls on omega-3 fatty acids, renowned for their heart-healthy properties and now celebrated for their role in keeping your brain sharp and resilient. Recent studies have illuminated the profound impact of fatty fish intake on mental acuity, underlining the importance of including these nutrient-rich options in your diet. Even when fresh fish isn't readily available, canned tuna, salmon, and sardines can become potent allies in nurturing your brain health. These omega-3 fatty acids represent a bridge between your physical well-being and your cognitive vitality, highlighting the intricate relationship between the foods you consume and the aging process.

As science continues its relentless march forward, the future promises personalized diets tailored to your unique genetic blueprint. Until that day arrives, we have the privilege of relishing the wealth of knowledge available today. As you unlock the secrets of these age-defying foods that nurture both body and mind, you embark on a journey toward a healthier, more vibrant, and fulfilling life

Chapter 6: Radiant Skin from Within: Nourishing Your Super Skin

Nourishing Your Skin: Beyond Surface Beauty

The age-old adage "we are what we eat" takes on profound significance when it comes to our skin, our body's largest and most visible organ. Often overlooked in our quest for beauty, our skin yearns for the tender care that proper nutrition can provide. Let's embark on a transformative journey into the world of skincare, where radiant, glowing skin is not merely a surface attribute but a reflection of the nourishment we provide from within.

Vitamin A: The Cornerstone of Skin Health

At the very core of skin health lies vitamin A, a nutrient that we simply cannot afford to overlook. Low-fat dairy products, such as yogurt, shine as some of the finest sources of this vital nutrient. Remarkably, low-fat yogurt not only abounds in vitamin A but also harbors acidophilus, those "live" bacteria that bolster intestinal health. What's even more intriguing is that their benevolent influence may extend to our skin. However, vitamin A isn't confined to the dairy aisle alone; it also resides in a diverse range of foods, including cod liver oil, sweet potatoes, carrots, leafy greens, and fortified breakfast cereals, all extending their skin-nourishing embrace.

Antioxidants: Nature's Guardians of Skin Cells

But the journey of skincare doesn't end with vitamin A alone; it beckons us to embrace the protective power of antioxidants. Fruits like blackberries, blueberries, strawberries, and plums, laden with antioxidants and phytochemicals, stand as stalwart guardians of our precious skin cells, shielding them from the ravages of oxidative stress. The result? Skin that ages gracefully, defying the relentless march of time. Joining this protective chorus are artichokes, beans, prunes, pecans, and an array of fruits and vegetables, each offering a vibrant spectrum of nutrients that contribute to the skin's vitality.

Essential Fatty Acids (EFAs): Champions of Cell Health

Essential fatty acids (EFAs) assume their vital role in skin health, and we invite salmon, walnuts, canola oil, and flax seeds to take center stage. EFAs champion the health of cell membranes, facilitating the passage of essential nutrients that nurture and sustain our skin. Equally crucial are healthy oils, such as cold-pressed olive or extra virgin oil, which bestow upon our skin the gift of lubrication and an enduring glow.

Selenium: Orchestrator of Skin Vitality

Selenium now enters the spotlight, a nutrient that orchestrates the well-being of our skin cells. From whole-wheat bread and muffins to turkey, tuna, and the mighty Brazil nuts, selenium's presence invigorates our skin's vitality. Recent studies hint at its remarkable potential, even in shielding sun-damaged skin from harm.

Complex Carbohydrates: Regulating Insulin for Clear Skin

Skincare is not merely an external pursuit; it delves deeper into our dietary choices. Opting for whole grains in complex carbohydrates can deftly regulate insulin levels, diminishing the specter of skin breakouts that haunt many. Green tea emerges as a soothing elixir, with anti-inflammatory prowess and a shield for cellular membranes, potentially curbing skin cancer risks.

Hydration: The Elixir of Youthful Vitality

And let's not forget the quintessential elixir of life: water. Its influence extends far beyond quenching our thirst. Well-hydrated skin, a testament to the body's inner harmony, radiates youthful vitality. Moreover, water undertakes the noble mission of purging toxins from our system, reducing their potential to wreak havoc and leaving our skin with a clear and radiant canvas.

In your pursuit of skin that transcends mere aesthetics, consider that it begins within you, within your plate of vibrant, nutrient-rich foods. Your skin, a testament to your inner health, deserves this nourishing embrace. As you embark on this holistic journey of skincare, remember that true beauty radiates from within, and it starts with the choices you make for your health and well-being.

Chapter 7: Stress-Busters: Superfoods to Conquer Life's Challenges

Revitalize Your Day: Superfoods to Beat Stress

In the whirlwind of our daily lives, stress often feels like an unwelcome companion, impacting our physical, mental, emotional, and spiritual well-being. Whether it's the demands of work, juggling family activities, running a household, or dealing with personal and family matters, the weight of it all can be overwhelming. However, don't underestimate the power of simple steps, particularly when it comes to the foods you eat, in your battle against stress. Let's explore how these superfoods can help you revitalize your day and combat stress effectively.

Kickstart Your Day with the Right Choices

When life feels particularly challenging, it's essential to make wise dietary choices. Avoiding excessive caffeine and alcohol is a smart starting point. These stimulants and depressants can sap your energy and hinder your ability to cope with stress. Similarly, sugary foods should be consumed in moderation, as they can lead to energy spikes and crashes that align with your daily stressors.

However, there's a host of superfoods ready to provide you with the energy and nutrients needed to tackle stress head-on and regain your vitality.

Asparagus: Your Mood-Boosting Friend

Asparagus, rich in folic acid, is a fantastic mood enhancer. Folic acid and vitamin B work together to produce serotonin, a chemical that can uplift your mood, even on the toughest days. Incorporating asparagus into your meals not only adds flavor but also nourishes your emotional well-being.

Red Meat: A Stress-Relief Dinner Choice

Despite some negative perceptions, red meat can be a healthy dinner option for individuals and families dealing with stress. Beef is packed with iron, zinc, and B vitamins that not only boost your mood but also help maintain a positive outlook, crucial for facing life's pressures. For those seeking a healthier choice, discussing lean cuts with your local butcher can provide a balance between nutrition and taste, ensuring that your stress-relief dinner remains satisfying and nutritious.

Milk: Your Morning Resilience Elixir

Milk deserves its reputation as a nutritional ally. Loaded with calcium, protein, antioxidants, and vitamins B2 and B12, it supports strong bones and the regeneration of healthy cells. Start your day by pairing low-fat milk with a wholesome whole-grain cereal to equip yourself against the challenges ahead. Cottage cheese is another dairy champion; when combined with vitamin C-rich fruits, it boosts your defenses against the free radicals that can take over during stressful times. This delicious combination provides nutrition and a burst of energy to help you tackle the day ahead.

Almonds: Warriors Against Stress

Almonds play a significant role in combating stress. Packed with magnesium, zinc, vitamins B2, C, and E, and heart-healthy unsaturated fats, they are potent warriors against free radicals, known culprits associated with conditions like cancer and heart disease. These nutritional powerhouses offer a convenient and delicious way to manage your stress levels, empowering you to confront life's challenges with resilience and vigor.

As you navigate life's challenges, remember that your plate offers more than sustenance; it provides you with the tools to combat stress. Embrace these superfoods, and fortify yourself against the daily storms of life, revitalizing your day and nurturing your well-being from within.